Baking Cookbook

The Essential Guide to Baking Delicious and Healthy Recipes for Beginners or Advance

Bonnie Mills

The information in the following pages is broadly considered a truthful and accurate account of facts and as such, any inattention, use, or misuse of the information in question by the reader will render any resulting actions solely under their purview. There are no scenarios in which the publisher or the original author of this work can be in any fashion deemed liable for any hardship or damages that may befall them after undertaking information described herein.

Additionally, the information in the following pages is intended only for informational purposes and should thus be thought of as universal. As befitting its nature, it is presented without assurance regarding its prolonged validity or interim quality. Trademarks that are mentioned are done without written consent and can in no way be considered an endorsement from the trademark holder.

Table of Contents

Baked Lunch Recipes

Triple Cheese And Onion Muffins

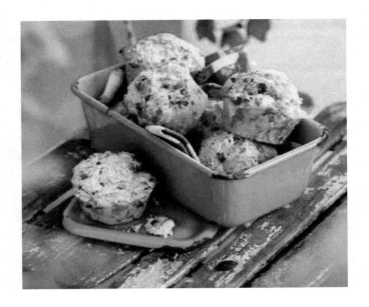

Prep Time: 15 minutes
Cook Time: 25 minutes
Servings: 12 people

Ingredients

- 1 cup of the extra virgin olive oil
- 1 golden egg
- 284 ml of buttermilk
- 3 cups of the all purpose flour
- 1 tablespoon of mustard powder
- 1 ½ cup of grated cheddar cheese
- 1 cup of the chopped spring onions
- 1 tablespoon of snipped chives
- ⅛ cup of the grated Parmesan cheese
- 2 cups of the soft cheese cut into cube shape

Directions

- Preheat an oven at 450 degrees F
- Take a muffin tray grease then with some olive oil. Take a bowl and add the egg, olive oil, and buttermilk. Whisk all the ingredients together until well combined
- Take another mixing bowl add flour, salt and mustard powder. Stir them together until well combined
- Then stir in them cheddar cheese, spring onions, chives and ½ of the parmesan cheese
- Now take a wooden spoon and fold the dry ingredients in the wet ingredients. Gently combine them. Then fold in them the soft cheese cubes
- Pour the mixture with the help of spoon on the muffin tins
- Scatter on them the remaining Parmesan cheese and then let them bake for about 25 minutes
- Then serve them and enjoy

Chicken, Apricot, And Pot Pie

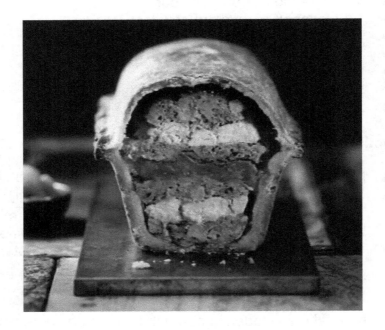

Prep Time: 2 hours
Cook Time: 1 hour and 30 minutes
Servings: 12 peoples

Ingredients

- 3 sausages of meat
- 250 grams of the dry rashers bacon roughly chopped
- 350 grams of the ham roughly chopped
- 1 tablespoon of the ground mace
- 1 tablespoon of the ground black pepper
- 4 tablespoons of the finely chopped parsley
- 400 grams of chicken fillets
- 20 soft and dry apricots
- 3 gelatin leaves
- 1 chicken stock cube
- 3 cups of all purpose flour
- 5 tablespoons of lard for greasing
- ⅛ cup of the milk
- 1 egg whisked together

Directions

- Preheat an oven at 450 degrees F
- Take a food processor add the sausage meat, ham, bacon, mace, pepper and some salt to taste.
- Pulse them until they are finely chopped
- Then carefully stir them in the pieces of ham and parsley
- Now make the pastries. Take a nonstick skillet and add flour, some salt, lard and milk, then add water, let them heat up on the low flame but don't overboil them
- Then pour this hot liquid in the flour mixture
- Let them heat with a wooden spoon
- Then pull out the dough and let them knead by using your hands for 10 minutes until it converts into smooth and elastic
- Now by using the lard grease the muffin tin. Then line them with the long strip of the greased parchment paper that comes out of the tin
- The dust some of the flour inside the tin. Put ⅓ of the dough in the tin then roll out to the rest of the roughly 1.5 cm thickness. Mold the pastry by using your hands

———

- Now start layering the pastry with the pork by pressing them with your hands, until they are firmly packed, even layer at the bottom
- Top them with half of the chicken strips, then with quarter of the pork. Repeat this process again and then top them with apricots
- Then fit them in snugly and once again create an even layer without no visible gap
- Then top them with half of the pork mixture over the apricots
- Then add the finely layer of the chicken fillets. Finely pile on the chicken fillets and mold on them by using neat until they are firmly done
- Now repeat this process with the rest of the pastries and brush them with eggs then press the top with the knife and let them bake for about 30 minutes
- Now put the gelatin leaves in the cold water to smooth them
- Then take a nonstick sauteing pan add hot water and chicken stock cube and stir them continuously then take out the leaves from the cold water and put them in the chicken stock
- Let them cool and insert the nozzle and pour the chicken stock in them. Then remove the nozzle and let them chill overnight
- Then serve them and enjoy

Smoked Salmon And Poppy Seed Palmier

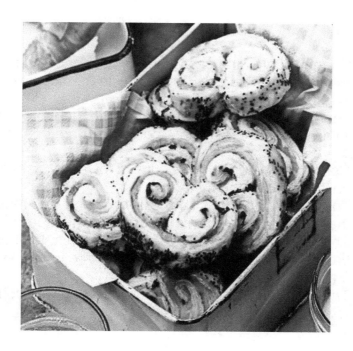

Prep Time: 25 minutes
Cook Time: 25 minutes
Servings: 12 people

Ingredients

- 350 grams of the puff pastry sheets
- 1 golden egg whisked together
- 1 tablespoon of the poppy seeds
- 5 tablespoons of the cream cheese
- 1 cup of the smoked salmon
- 1 small bunch of chopped snipped

Directions

- Carefully unroll the pastry and on one end brush them with the beaten eggs. Then sprinkle the poppy seeds and turn over the pastry
- Then spread over cream cheese and then top them with the smoked salmon. Then scatter on them over the chives
- Roll on them and fold the ends in towards the middle until you reach the centre
- Then cut in the slices into pieces. Then place them on the baking tray lined with the parchment paper
- Then transfer them to the baking oven and let them bake for about 25 minutes until they are turned into crispy and golden brown
- Then let them cool down and serve them with your favorite sauce and enjoy

Cheese And Marmite Scones

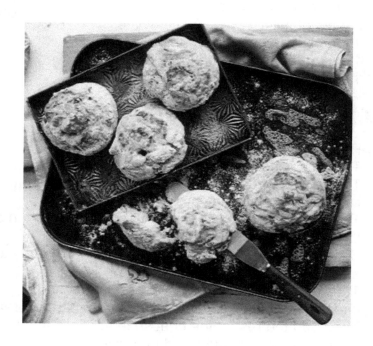

Prep Time: 20 minutes
Cook Time: 15 minutes
Servings: 12 people

Ingredients

- 3 cups of all purpose flour
- 1 tablespoon of the baking powder
- 3 tablespoons of the marinate
- 1 golden egg whisked
- 2 cups of milk
- 1 tablespoon of extra virgin olive oil
- 1 cup of the grated cheddar cheese
- 1 cup of the heavy whipping cream

Directions

- Preheat an oven at 450 degrees F
- Take a baking tray and spray them with some flour. Take a bowl, add flour, and baking flour. Stir them continuously until they are well combined
- Then take a jug add 1 tablespoon of marmite then add the egg, then make them to 300 ml of milk
- Stir them in oil and beat them until they are ready to dissolve the marmite
- Take a bowl add the cream cheese, and cheddar cheese and the remaining marmite to make a spread
- Then add the rest of the cheese in the flour and then pour in the milk mixture and then stir them with the spoon
- Pull out the dough on the floured surface and knead them for 10 minutes
- Then press them in the long shape and put them in the oblong shape pan. Then spread on them marimite and roll on them tightly, fat cylinder. Then pat the ends of the pastry to straighten them
- Then cut them in 8 pinwheels. Let them put them on the baking tray
- Then flatten them to make rounds
- Then bake them for about 15 minutes
- Then let them cool down and then set them aside
- Serve them and enjoy

Brie, Courgette And Red Pepper Muffins

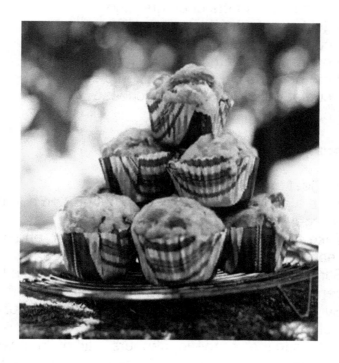

Prep Time: 25 minutes
Cook Time: 35 minutes
Servings: 10 people

Ingredients

- 1 tablespoon of the butter
- 2 small sized and 1 large courgetti (then cut them in small sized cubes)
- 2 cups of the all purpose flour
- 1 teaspoon of the baking powder
- 1 tablespoon of the fresh oregano leaves
- 1 tablespoon of the dried oregano
- 3 golden eggs beaten
- 1 cup of the milk
- 5 tablespoons of the extra virgin olive oil
- 2 red peppers cut into bite-sized pieces
- 1 cup of the grated cheddar cheese
- 1 cup camembert

Directions

- Preheat an oven at 450 degrees F
- Take a nonstick pan melt some butter then add the courgette let then cook for 5 minutes
- Take a bowl add the flour, baking powder, and some seasonings in a bowl
- Stir them to combine and then make the well in the centre and crack the golden eggs, milk and oil
- Stir them to combine all the ingredients together until well combined
- Then add the courgette, peppers, half of the cheddar cheese and all the brie or Camembert in the batter
- Stir them continuously until they are well combined. Pour this batter in an oil greased muffins tray and then let them bake for about 30 minutes until they are turned into golden brown and crispy
- Then serve them and enjoy

Classic Cheese Scones

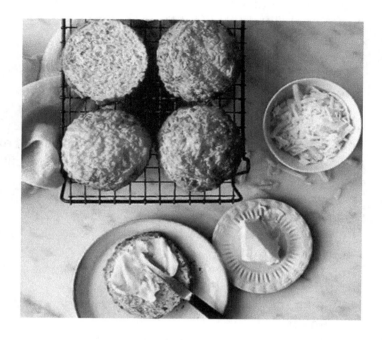

Prep Time: 15 minutes
Cook Time: 20 minutes
Servings: 6 people

Ingredients

- 3 cups of all purpose flour
- Some salt to taste
- Some ground black pepper to taste
- 1 teaspoon of baking soda
- ½ cup of chilled butter (cut them in cubes shape
- 2 cups of the grated cheddar cheese
- 1 ½ cups of milk

Directions

- Preheat an oven at 450 degrees F
- Take a bowl add the flour, salt, cayenne pepper, baking soda, into bowl mix all the ingredients together until well combined
- Then add the chilled butter and then combine them by using your fingers to make a breadcrumbs
- Then sprinkle the cheese in the pan spread that they are evenly distributed
- Then pour the milk in them to make a thick and elastic dough.
- Then take out the dough and roll on them to make a thick sheet
- Take out the cutter and then cut out the scones by using it
- Then put them on the baking sheet lined with parchment paper. Spray some oil brush them with egg and then sprinkle the cheese on them
- Then transfer the baking tray in the oven and let them bake for about 20 minutes until it turns into golden brown and crispy

Cheesy Sausage Rolls

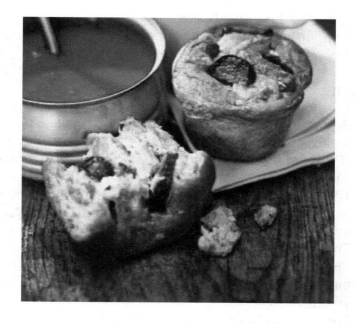

Prep Time: 1 hour 20 minutes
Cook Time: 1 hour 50 minutes
Servings: 12 people

Ingredients

- 3 cups of the bread mix (package or ready made)
- Some oil for greasing
- 8 sausages cooked
- Some cornmeal for dusting
- ½ cup of the garlic butter
- 6 spring onions finely chopped
- 2 cups of the grated Parmesan cheese

Directions

- Preheat an oven at 450 degrees F
- Make a bread mix by following the package instructions
- Then set them aside for some time in warm place until it is risen or doubled
- Take a nonstick pan and grease them with some olive oil. Put the cooked sausages in the pan and again heat up them for 1 minute
- Then remove them and cut them in 1cm slices
- Then pull out the dough out of the bowl and then knead them for about 10 minutes until they are elastic or smooth
- Then roll on them in the rectangular size
- Then brush the dough with the garlic butter and scatter some spring onions, cheese and sausages
- Now roll up the dough like a swiss roll. Then use a sharp knife and cut them into 12 pieces
- Take a muffin tray and brush them with some melted butter. Then put the swiss rolls bread cut side up into each hole. Then dap the remaining butter over there tops and then close them with an oiled cling film
- Then set them aside for 30 minutes
- Transfer the pan to the oven and let them bake for about 25 minutes until it turns into golden brown and crispy
- Then remove them from the oven and enjoy

Cheese And Marinate Pasties

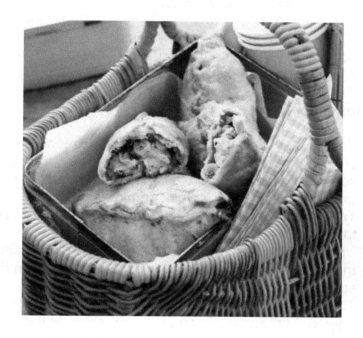

Prep Time: 25 minutes
Cook Time: 1 hour
Servings: 6 people

Ingredients

- 3 cups of peeled and grated potatoes
- 2 cups of the grated cheddar cheese
- 1 cup of breadcrumbs
- 3 spring onions finely chopped
- 2 golden eggs
- 500 grams of the short crust pastry
- Some all purpose flour for dusting
- 2 tablespoons of the marmite

Directions

- Take a bowl add the grated potatoes, cheese, breadcrumbs and spring onions. Then add the egg, sprinkle some salt and black pepper. Then stir them together until they are well combined
- Take out the pastry sheets and then roll on them like a thick coin
- Use a pastry cutter and cut the circles. Take a bowl add the marmite and then add the splash of water on then so that it has less consistency
- Then brush them on the circles then spread the beaten eggs on the edges. Then pinch the sides of the pastries. Then transfer the pastries to the baking oven and then bake them for about 50 minutes until it turns into golden brown and crispy
- Then serve them and enjoy

Leek, Goat Cheese, Walnut And Lemon Tart

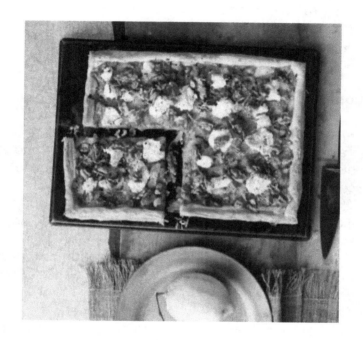

Prep Time: 25 minutes
Cook Time: 30 minutes
Servings: 4 people

Ingredients

- 1 tablespoon of extra virgin olive oil
- ⅛ cup of the melted butter
- 2 medium sized leeks sliced
- 3 tablespoons of the thyme leaves
- 1 tablespoon of lemon juice
- 1 tablespoons of lemon zest
- 375 grams of ready rolled puff pastry
- 2 cups of hand torn goat cheese
- ½ cup of the walnuts chopped
- Some finely chopped parsley

Directions

- Preheat an oven at 450 degree F
- Take nonstick pan add olive oil in them then add the butter, once it starts sizzling then add the leek let them cook until they are tendered
- Then add the thyme leaves, lemon juice, lemon zest, increase the heat. Let them cook and sprinkle some salt and ground black pepper
- Now lay the pastry sheet on the baking sheet lined with the parchment paper. Lightly mark the edges of the pastry sheet with the fork
- Then slightly prick the whole bread sheet
- Then spread them leeks on the pastry sheet. Then crumble the cheese and walnuts then sprinkle some salt and black pepper
- Drizzle some olive oil. Then put the tart in the oven and let them bake for about 15 minutes until the pastry puffs and it turns into golden brown and crispy
- Then scatter the with the lemon zest on the top
- Then serve them and enjoy

Cheese And Caramelized Onion Coburg

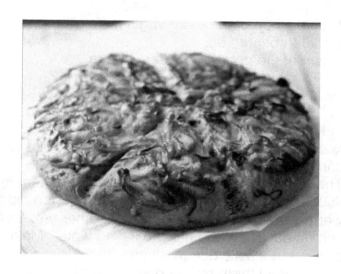

Prep Time: 20 minutes
Cook Time: 30 minutes
Servings: 4 people

Ingredients

- 3 cups of the grain bread flour
- 1 cup of the wheat bread flour
- 2 tablespoons of the dry nutritional yeast
- Some salt to taste
- Someone ground black pepper to taste
- 1 tablespoon of the softened butter
- 1 large sized onion cut into wedges
- 1 tablespoon of the extra virgin olive oil
- 1 golden beaten eggs
- ½ cup of the grated cheddar cheese

Directions

- Take a bowl add all the flours, yeast and salt. Stir them to combine all the ingredients together until well combined
- Then put the butter in them and then rub them in the flour. Then stir them in a flour mixture. Then dip the warm water and then mix them together until well combined. Then add the remaining water. Make a sticky and elastic dough. Gather them in the bowl
- Then knead them by using your hands until it is elastic and smooth
- Then put the dough on the lightly floured surface covered with a damp kitchen towel for 2 hours
- After 2 hours pull the dough out of the oven and cut them in 2 balls then flatten then in round shape
- Put the round dough shape on the lightly floured surface lined with the parchment paper greased with some oil, brush them with some egg wash, scatter the onions, then sprinkle the grated cheese
- Transfer the baking pan in the oven and let them bake for about 20 minutes
- Then after 20 minutes pour the water on the tin and again bake them for about 35 minutes until it turns golden into brown and crispy
- Then remove them and serve

- Enjoy

Chorizo And Mozzarella Bake

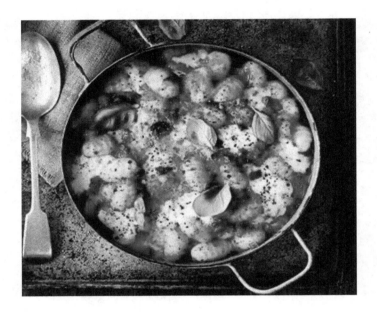

Prep Time: 10 minutes
Cook Time: 25 minutes
Servings: 6 people

Ingredients

- 1 tablespoon of the extra virgin olive oil
- 1 small sized onion grated
- 2 minced garlic cloves
- 1 ½ cups of chorizo in diced form
- 2 cans of the chopped tomatoes
- 1 tablespoon of the caster sugar
- 3 cups of the fresh gnocchi
- 1 ½ cups of the mozzarella cheese cut into cube sized
- ½ cup the chopped basil leaves
- Some green salad for serving

Directions

- Take a nonstick pan and drizzle in some olive oil. Then put the finely chopped onions and minced garlic. Let them sauté for about 10 minutes until they are soft or tendered
- Then add the chorizo and let them cook for about 5 minutes
- Then put in them chopped tomatoes, sugar and sprinkle some salt and black pepper to taste
- Let them simmer and add the gnocchi and let them cook for about 8 minutes
- Then stir the mozzarella and some of the chopped basil leaves over them
- Let them cook for about 3 minutes. Then divide the mixture over 6 ramekins then sprinkle some more mozzarella then transfer them to the baking oven at 450 degrees F for about 5 minutes until the cheese starts melting
- Season them with some salt and black pepper and sprinkle some basil leaves. Then serve them with green salad
- Serve them and enjoy

Easy Butter Chicken

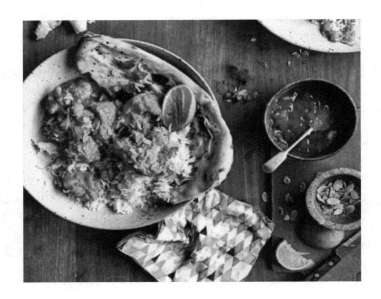

Prep Time: 15 minutes
Cook Time: 35 minutes
Servings: 4 people

Ingredients

- 500 grams of the boneless and skinless chicken breasts.

For the marinade

- 2 tablespoons of the lemon juice
- 2 tablespoons of the ground cumin seeds
- 2 tablespoons of the smoked paprika
- 1 teaspoon of the hot chili powder
- 2 cups of the natural yoghurt

For the curry

- 2 tablespoons of the extra virgin olive oil
- 1 large onion finely chopped
- 3 minced garlic cloves
- 1 large sized green chili deseeded, and finely chopped
- 1 tablespoon of the grated ginger
- 1 tablespoon of the whole spice powder
- 2 tablespoons of the fenugreek powder
- 3 tablespoons of the tomato puree
- 2 cups of the chicken stock
- 4 tablespoons of the flaked almonds (toasted)
- 1 bowl of the boil rice
- 1 wheat bread
- Someone lemon wedges
- Lime pickle
- Freshly chopped parsley

Directions

- Take a bowl and add all the marinade ingredients in them, season them with some salt and black pepper. Then chop the chicken into bite-sized chunks and then dip them in the bowl
- Then let them marinade for about 2 hours. Till then nonstick sauteing pan add the olive oil, add the onions,

garlic, green chili and ginger. Sprinkle some salt and black pepper to taste
- Then let them heat for 10 minutes until they are softened
- Then add the tomato puree then let them cook for 2 minutes
- Then add the chicken stock and marinated chicken
- Then let then cool for about 10 minutes. Then add the remaining marinade in the pan. Let them simmer for about 5 minutes. Then sprinkle some roasted almonds on them
- Serving them with rice, bread, lime wedges and lime pickle
- Serve them and enjoy

Easy Classic Lasagne

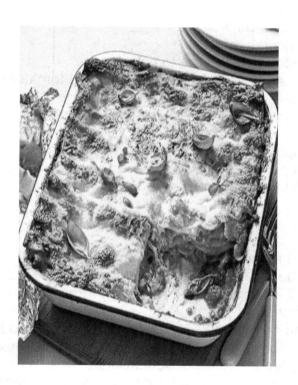

Prep Time: 15 minutes
Cook Time: 60 minutes
Servings: 6 people

Ingredients

- 1 tablespoon of the extra virgin olive oil
- 3 rashers of the smoked streaky bacon
- 1 large onion finely chopped
- 1 celery stick finely chopped
- 1 small carrot grated
- 2 minced garlic cloves
- 2 minced beef
- 2 tablespoons of the tomato puree
- 2 cans of cans of the finely chopped tomatoes
- 1 tablespoon of honey
- 500 grams of the fresh egg lasagna sheets
- 400 ml of the creme fraiche
- 2 cups of the hand torn mozzarella cheese
- ⅛ cup of the grated Parmesan cheese
- Hand full of the torn basil leaves

Directions

- Take a nonstick sauteing pan add some olive oil. Cut the bacon strips and then put them in the pan let them cook for about 5 minutes until it turns into golden brown and crispy
- Then add the onions, celery and carrots and let them cook for about 5 minutes while stirring occasionally until they are tendered or softened
- Then add the minced garlic stir them and break them for 2 minutes until they are turned into golden brown
- Then pour the tomato puree and let them cook for about 2 minutes. Then add the minced beef and vegetables
- Then add the chopped tomatoes
- Let them cook while continuously stirring then sprinkle some salt and black pepper. Add the honey
- The let them simmer for about 5 minutes
- Preheat an oven at 450 degrees F
- Now take a casserole dish, assemble the lasagna, ladle a little of the ragu sauce in the bottom

- Then spread the sauce all over the base
- Then put 2 sheets of the lasagna on the top of the sauce and add another layer of the pasta
- Then repeat this process
- Now take a bowl add the creme fraiche in a bowl and then add some water to make a thick sauce
- Then pour this sauce on the top of the pasta and then sprinkle the mozzarella cheese. Pour this sauce on the pasta
- Then again top them with the mozzarella cheese
- Transfer the pan to the oven and then let them bake for about 30 minutes until the cheese starts melting and bubbling
- Then serve the and enjoy

Thai Fried Prawn And Pineapple Rice

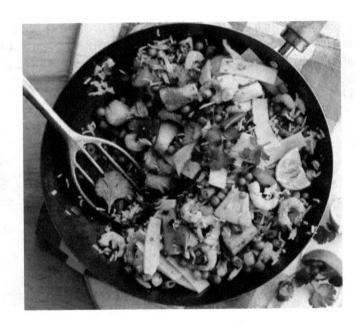

Prep Time: 10 minutes
Cook Time: 15 minutes
Servings: 4 people

Ingredients

- 2 tablespoons of extra virgin olive oil
- 1 cup of onions, (green, white and red finely chopped)
- 1 large sized green chili deseeded and finely chopped into chunks
- 1 cup of the pineapple (cut into chunk sized)
- 3 tablespoons of the Thai green curry sauce
- 4 tablespoons of the soy sauce
- 2 cups of the brown rice uncooked
- 2 golden eggs whisked together
- ½ cup of the frozen peas
- 225 grams of the bamboo shoots, drained
- 2 cups of the frozen prawns, cooked and raw
- 1 tablespoon of the lemon juice
- Some lemon wedges
- 1 tablespoon of the chopped coriander leaves for garnishing

Directions

- Take a nonstick pan add the olive oil let them heat up then add the onions let them cook for about 2 minutes until they are tendered or softened
- Then stir in then peppers, pineapples, soy sauce and curry paste. Let them cook for about 5 minutes
- Then add the water-soaked rice, stir them frequently until they are piping out
- Then lightly push the eggs to one side and the scrambled eggs to the other side
- Then stir in them the peas, bamboo shoots, and prawns into the eggs and rice
- Let them cook for about 5 minutes
- Then finely stir in them spring green onions, lime juice and coriander
- Then transfer them in a bowl and then serve them with lime wedges
- And then serve them with sauce sauce
- Serve then and enjoy

One Pan Spaghetti With Nduja, Fennel And Olives

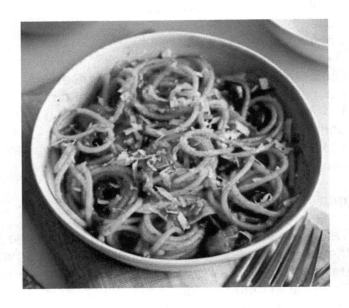

Prep Time: 15 minutes
Cook Time: 15 minutes
Servings: 4 people

Ingredients

- 2 cups of the spaghetti
- 3 minced garlic cloves
- 1 fennel halved and thinly sliced
- 80 grams of nduja paste
- 2 cans of the tomatoes chopped and chunked
- ⅛ cup of the black olives pitted and sliced
- 3 tablespoons of the tomato puree
- 3 tablespoons of extra virgin olive oil
- 2 tablespoons of the red wine vinegar
- 40 grams of the pecorino
- Handful of the chopped basil leaves

Directions

- Take a deep frying pan add all the ingredients except pecorino, and basil leaves
- Deep fry them and sprinkle some salt and black pepper. Pour the hot water over them and let them simmer and let the spaghetti soften
- Then let then simmer for about 12 minutes
- Then stir them through the pecorino, and basil leaves
- Then serve them with a drizzle of some olive oil and pecorino on the side
- Enjoy

Easy Chicken Fajitas

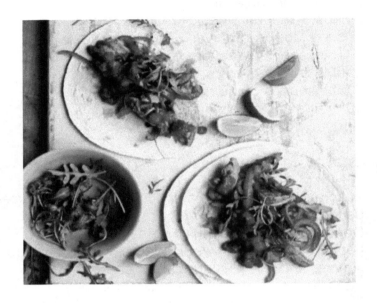

Prep Time: 15 minutes
Cook Time: 10 minutes
Servings: 3 people

Ingredients

- 2 large sized chicken breasts finely sliced
- 1 large onion finely chopped
- 1 red bell pepper finely sliced
- 1 large sized red chili finely sliced
- 1 tablespoon of the smoked paprika
- 1 tablespoon of the ground cumin powder
- 1 tablespoon of the coriander powder
- 2 minced garlic cloves
- 1 tablespoon of the lemon juice
- 4 drops of the Tabasco
- Tortillas
- Some salad to serve
- Some fresh salsa

Directions

- Preheat an oven at 450 degrees
- Wrap the 6 tortillas in foil
- Take a bowl add the smoked paprika, ground coriander, ground cumin, minced garlic cloves, olive oil, lemon juice, 4 drops of Tabasco. Sprinkle salt and black pepper stir them to combine all the ingredients together until well combined
- Then add the sliced chicken pieces and then finely chopped onions, finely chopped red pepper and then red chili. Stir them to combine well and then coat them
- Take a deep sauteing pan, then add the marinated chicken let them cook on high heat for 5 minutes until you get nice charred effects
- Then put the rolled tortillas on the chicken pieces. Let them cook for about 5 minutes
- Then add the mixed salad and then tub of the fresh salsa
- Then serve them and enjoy

Easy Carrot Cake

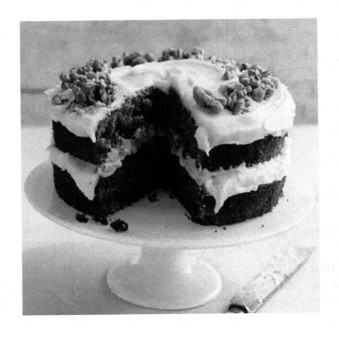

Prep Time: 35 minutes
Cook Time: 30 minutes
Servings: 12 people

Ingredients

- 5 tablespoons of extra virgin olive oil
- ½ cup of the yogurt
- 4 golden eggs
- 2 tablespoons vanilla extract
- 1 tablespoon of the orange zest
- 2 cups of the all purpose flour
- ½ cup of the light muscovado sugar
- 2 tablespoons of the ground cinnamon
- 2 tablespoons of the fresh nutmeg finely grated
- 3 small grated carrots
- 100 grams of the sultanas
- ¼ cup of pecan And walnuts roughly chopped
- ½ cup of the unsalted butter softened
- 5 tablespoons of the icing sugar
- ¼ cup of the soft cheese

Directions

- Preheat an oven at 450 degrees F
- Take a cake pan lined with the parchment paper and grease them with some olive oil
- Take a bowl add oil, yogurt, eggs, vanilla extract, orange zest, flour, sugar, nutmeg with some salt. Stir them together by using your fingers
- Then add the grated carrots, raisins and half of the nuts. If you are using then mix them together until well combined
- Pour this batter in the cake pan and then let them bake for about 30 minutes
- Take a bowl add the sugar and butter let them combine well
- Then remove the cake from the tin and then top with the icing and then sprinkle the chopped walnuts
- Then set them aside for about 2 hours until they are chilled
- Then serve them and enjoy

Piri-Piri Chicken With Mashed Sweet Potatoes And Broccoli

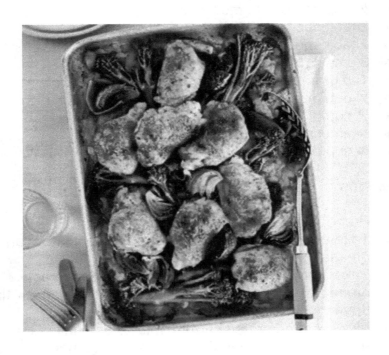

Prep Time: 20 minutes
Cook Time: 25 minutes
Servings: 3 people

Ingredients

- 3 large sweet potato (peeled and cut into chunk)
- 1 tablespoon extra virgin olive oil
- 8 chicken thighs skin on
- 2 large red onion, cut into wedges
- 2 tablespoons of the piri spice mix
- 2 cups of the long stem broccoli

Directions

- Preheat an oven at 450 degrees F
- Take a large tin, add the sweet potatoes chunks sprinkle some salt and pepper and then olive oil. Toss them to combine all the ingredients together until well combined
- Push the potatoes to one end of the tin and the chicken with onions to the other side, then sprinkle some spices, drizzle some oil and some seasonings
- Now transfer them to the oven and let them roast for about 40 minutes while stirring them halfway through
- Then put the broccoli, then drizzle with some oil and season them
- Let them roast for about 15 minutes
- Remove the onions, chicken and broccoli from the tin. Then mash the potatoes by using fork
- Put the mashed potatoes in a plate. Then top them with the chicken, broccoli and onions
- Then serve them and enjoy

Easy Meatballs

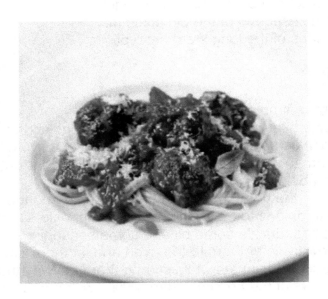

Prep Time: 1 hour
Cook Time: 40 minutes
Servings: 4 people

Ingredients

- 400 grams of the good quality pork sausage
- 1 small sized onion finely chopped
- 1 small carrot grated
- 1 tablespoon of the dried oregano
- 2 cups of the lean minced beef
- ⅓ cup of the grated Parmesan cheese
- ¼ cup of the dried breadcrumbs
- 1 large golden egg
- 1 tablespoon of the extra virgin olive oil
- 1 small carrot finely grated
- 2 celery sticks finely grated
- 1 courgette finely grated
- 2 red peppers
- 3 minced garlic cloves
- 2 red pepper finely chopped
- 1 tablespoon of the extra virgin olive oil
- 2 tablespoons of the tomato puree
- Some pinch of caster sugar
- ½ teaspoon of the red wine vinegar
- ¼ cup of the finely chopped tomatoes
- 1 bowl of the cooked spaghetti
- Handful of the chopped basil leaves

Directions

- Take a bowl add the sausage meat our of the skin, drizzle some olive oil
- Then finely grate the onions, and carrots. The finely grate the Parmesan cheese, vegetables and garlic and then set them aside
- Now take a meatball ingredients in the bowl and add the rest of the ingredients. Then mix all the ingredients with your hands
- Then make the meatballs by using your hands and then put them in the tray then cover then with the cling film and have a little tidy up
- Now take peppers and remove the seeds and then cut

the peppers in half sized

- Take a large sauteing pan, add the olive oil, then aesthetically vegetables and garlic let them cook for about 5 minutes
- Then add tomatoes puree, sugar, vinegar, let them cook for about 2 minutes then add the chopped tomatoes in then let them simmer for about 5 minutes
- Blend the sauce by using the wooden spoon. Then let the sauce simmer
- Take a nonstick pan add some olive oil then put the meatballs. Then let them brown from both sides
- Then put the sauce in the batches, let them simmer for about 15 minutes while stirring until they are cooked through
- Top them with the grated Parmesan cheese and hand torn basil leaves
- Then serve them with the spaghetti
- Serve them and enjoy

Easy Beef Hot Pot

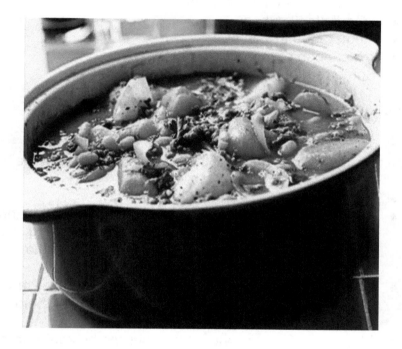

Prep Time: 45 minutes
Cook Time: 45 minutes
Servings: 6 people

Ingredients

- 2 large onions finely diced
- 3 small sized carrots grated
- 1 kilo potatoes in diced form
- 2 cups of lean minced beef
- 2 beef stock cubes
- 1 cup of the frozen beans
- 1 teaspoon of the Worcheshire sauce
- Some roughly chopped parsley for garnishing

Directions

- Take a bowl, add the onions and cut them into 8 wedges. Roughly chop the carrots and then cut the potatoes into chunks
- Then out the kettle on the flame
- Take a nonstick pan, add the extra virgin olive oil and minced garlic and let them fry them, while stirring occasionally until they are tendered or turned into golden brown
- Then crumble the chicken stock cubes and then mix them. Add the prepared veggies and then stir them occasionally
- Then pour the hot water, then pour the hot water from the kettle. Bring them to boil
- Then let them simmer for about 30 minutes
- Then stir the baked beans in them and pour the Worcheshire sauce, let them heat
- Sprinkle some salt and black pepper stir them occasionally until they are well combined
- Scatter the chopped parsley, then put them in the bowls then serve them and enjoy

Unbelievable Easy Mince Pie

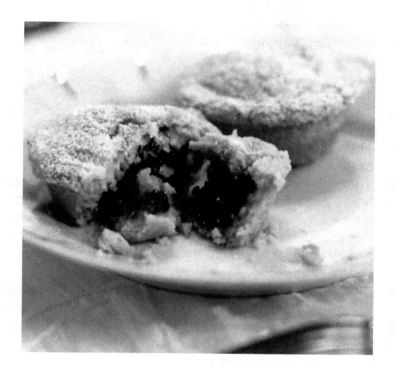

Prep Time: 25 minutes
Cook Time: 40 minutes
Servings: 12 people

Ingredients

- 1 cup of the cold butter
- 2 cups of the all purpose flour
- ⅛ cup of the caster sugar
- 2 cups of the minced meat
- 1 small egg beaten
- Some icing sugar to dust

Directions

- Take a bowl add the flour, butter, caster sugar, and some salt
- Then combine the pastry in a bowl, then knead them briefly. Knead the dough for about 5 minutes
- Then preheat an oven at 450 degrees F. Then take 12 holes patty tins and then press the dough in the tin holes
- Put the minced beef in each party sheet. Take another pastry sheet and put on the minced beef and make pies by using your hands
- Then top the pastries edges with the lids by pressing the edges to seal them
- Then brush the top of the pies with the beaten eggs
- Let them bake for about 20 minutes until they are turned into crispy and golden brown
- Then remove them on the rack and sprinkle some icing sugar
- Then serve them and enjoy

Frying Pan Pizza With Aubergine, Ricotta And Mint

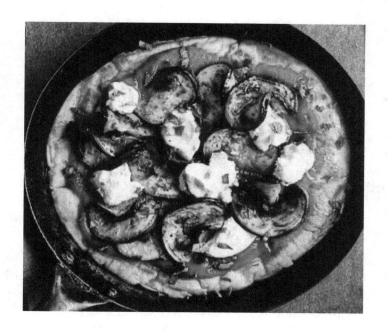

Prep Time: 25 minutes
Cook Time: 35 minutes
Servings: 4 people

Ingredients

- 2 cups of the all purpose flour
- 1 tablespoon of dry nutritional yeast
- ½ teaspoon of the caster sugar
- Some extra olive oil for greasing

Toppings

- 4 tablespoons of the extra virgin olive oil
- 1 tablespoon of the minced garlic cloves
- 1 cup of the passata
- ⅛ tablespoon of the caster sugar
- 1 small of the aubergine (sliced into discs)
- ½ cup of the ricotta
- ⅛ cup of the chopped mint leaves
- Someone extra virgin olive for drizzling

Directions

- Take a bowl add flour, lukewarm water, yeast, salt, oil and caster sugar. Stir them to combine all the ingredients together until well combined
- Until the thick and elastic dough is formed, then pull the dough out of the bowl and then knead them for 5 minutes until the dough is thick and elastic
- Then put the dough in the bowl and cover them with a damp kitchen towel and let them set aside for 2 hours
- Take a bowl add all the sauce ingredients and stir them to combine well. Then take a bowl add the olive oil and pour the sauce ingredients in the pan and let them cook for about 10 minutes
- Let them simmer. Then add some caster sugar and let them too tart. Set them aside
- Take out the pizza dough and roll on them in round pizza shape
- Then put the pizza dough in the pan. Brush the surface of the dough with some extra virgin olive oil and then sprinkle the cling film

---

- Then set them aside for 15 minutes until they are doubled
- Take a nonstick pan, add the olive oil, then add the aubergine in the pan. Then sprinkle some salt and black pepper. Then let them cook for 5 minutes. Let them cook and then transfer them to the bowl and then cover them with a foil to keep them warm
- Take a nonstick pan add some olive oil then carefully put the dough in the pan, let them cook until they are turned into golden brown and hard
- Flip them a little and drizzle some olive oil on the edges.
- Let them cook for about 5 minutes more
- Then spread the sauce over the dough evenly. Top them with some aubergines and some ricotta. Sprinkle the mint leaves and then drizzle some extra virgin olive oil
- Then serve them and enjoy

Easy Millionmaire's Short Bread

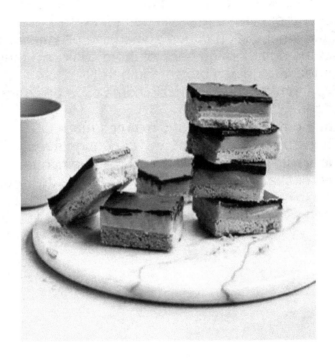

Prep Time: 25 minutes
Cook Time: 35 minutes
Servings: 24 people

Ingredients

- 3 cups of all purpose flour
- ¼ cup of caster sugar
- 1 cup of the unsalted or softened butter
- ¼ cup of the butter or margarine
- ¼ cup of the light muscovado sugar
- 1 ½ cans of the condensed milk
- 2 cups of the broken chocolate

Directions

- Preheat an oven at 350 degrees F
- Take a rectangular baking pan lined with the parchment paper and grease then with some olive oil, take a bowl add flour caster sugar, unsalted butter, then rub them in softened butter (until they are converted into fine breadcrumbs)
- Then pull out the dough and knead them until it is elastic and smooth
- Take out the rolling pin and roll the dough in rectangular shape
- Then let them prick with a fork
- Let then bake for about 20 minutes until it turns into golden brown and crispy
- Take a nonstick pan add the butter, margarine, muscovado sugar and condensed milk. Let then simmer on low flame. Let them heat up until it is dissolved and is converted into thick liquid
- Pour this on the shortbread and let then cool.
- Then take a nonstick pan add the chocolate pieces and let them melt on low flame until it is melted
- Then put this on the cold caramel and then set them aside
- Then cut them in the hot bars and serve them and enjoy

Easy Huevos Rancheros

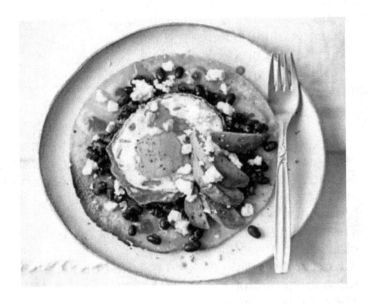

Prep Time: 3 minutes
Cook Time: 7 minutes
Servings: 4 people

Ingredients

- 1 tablespoon of the extra virgin olive oil
- 1 corn tortilla wrap
- 1 golden egg
- 1 can of the black beans drained
- 1 tablespoon of the extra virgin olive oil
- ½ ripe of the avocados peeled and sliced
- ⅓ cup of the crumbled feta cheese
- 2 tablespoons of the hot sauce

Directions

- Take a nonstick pan sprinkle some olive oil then heat up the corn tortillas until it turns into crispy and golden brown
- Then transfer them to the pan, cook the egg, then take a bowl, add the beans into the bowl and sprinkle some salt and black pepper. Then pour the lemon juice. Mash them by using fork
- Then transfer the beans to the tortillas and then top them with an egg, avocado slices, feta and chili sauce
- Squeeze some lemon juice and then serve them and enjoy

Vegetarian Chilli

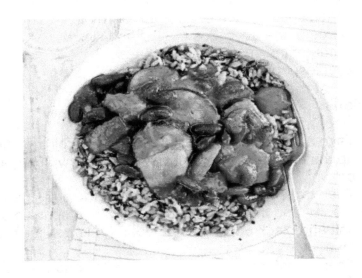

Prep Time: 2 minutes
Cook Time: 30 minutes
Servings: 4 people

Ingredients

- 2 cups of the roasted vegetables
- 1 can of the kidney beans dipped in chili sauce
- 1 can of the chopped tomatoes
- ⅓ cup of the ready-to-eat mixed grain
- Some salt to taste
- Some ground black pepper to taste

Directions

- Preheat an oven at 450 degrees F
- Take a baking dish grease them with some olive oil put the vegetables in a casserole dish let them bake for about 15 minutes
- Then put the beans, tomatoes, sprinkle some salt and black pepper to taste and let them cook for another 15 minutes
- Then remove them and serve with chili

Easy treacle Sponge

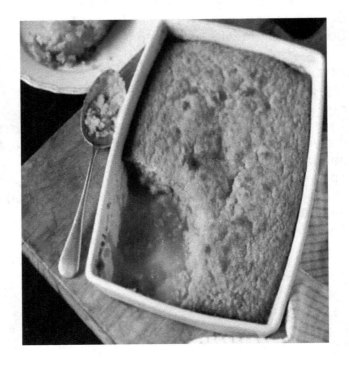

Prep Time: 15 minutes
Cook Time: 40 minutes
Servings: 8 people

Ingredients

- 1 cup of the golden syrup
- 1 tablespoon of lemon zest
- 1 tablespoon of the lemon juice
- ¼ cup of the breadcrumbs
- ½ cup of the softened butter
- ⅓ cup of the caster sugar
- 3 golden eggs
- 2 cups of the self raising flour
- 5 tablespoons of the milk

Directions

- Preheat an oven at 450 degrees F
- Take a bowl and add the golden syrup, lemon zest, lemon juice, breadcrumbs. Stir them to combine all the ingredients together until well combined
- Then spread this mixture in the baking dish
- Take a bowl egg the eggs, butter, sugar. Let then beat until they are fluffy then stir them in the milk and flour and then dollop over the syrup
- Transfer them to the baking oven and then let them bake for about 40 minutes until it turns into golden brown and crispy
- Then serve with lots of custard, cream, ice cream and extra dripple of syrup
- Then serve them and enjoy

Easy Rocky Road

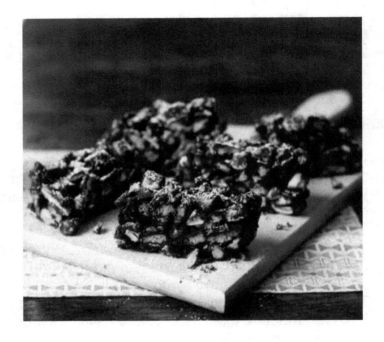

Prep Time: 15 minutes
Cook Time: 5 minutes
Servings: 12 people

Ingredients

- 2 cups of the digestive biscuits
- 1 cup of the unsalted melted butter
- 2 cups of the dark chocolate
- 3 tablespoons of the golden syrup
- 1 cup of the chopped marshmallows
- Some icing sugar to sprinkle
- ⅓ cup of the dried cranberries
- 2 tablespoons of the nuts
- ¼ cup of popcorn
- ⅛ cup of the honeycomb broken into pieces

Directions

- Preheat and oven at 459 degrees F
- Take a square brownie tin, lined with the parchment paper and grease them with some olive oil
- Take digestive biscuits put them in the bag and roll on them by using rolling pin and crash them into fine lumps or breadcrumbs
- Then set them aside
- Take a nonstick pan melt the butter, golden syrup and then stir them on low flame until well combined
- Then set them aside and let them cool down
- Take a bowl add the biscuits, chopped marshmallows, dried fruits, nuts, popcorn, and honeycombs. Then stir them together until well combined and then pour them in the chocolate mixture
- Then stir them until well combined
- Pour this mixture in the baking tin and spread them with the spoon.
- Let them freeze for 3 hours and then sprinkle some icing sugar on the top
- Then cut them into 12 fingers

Easy Chicken Tagine

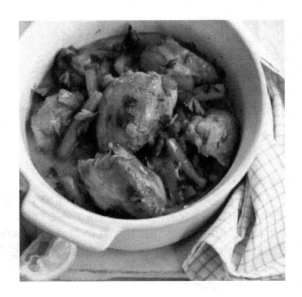

Prep Time: 10 minutes
Cook Time: 40 minutes
Servings: 4 people

Ingredients

- 2 tablespoons of extra virgin olive oil
- 8 skinless and boneless chicken breast
- 1 large onion finely chopped
- 2 tablespoons of the finely grated ginger
- Some turmeric to sprinkle
- Some saffron to sprinkle
- 1 tablespoon of honey
- 2 cups of the carrots cut into sticks
- 1 bunch of finely chopped parsley
- Some lemon wedges to top

Directions

- Take a nonstick pan sprinkle some oil and put the chicken thighs on them and then let them cook from both sides
- Until they changed their color
- Then add the ginger, and onion let then fry for about 3 minutes
- Then add water, saffron, honey, and carrots. Sprinkle some salt and black pepper then stir them to combine well. Let them simmer for about 30 minutes until the chicken is tendered
- Then increase the flame for about 5 minutes
- Sprinkle some chopped parsley and some lemon wedges
- Then serve them and enjoy

Easy Chicken Kiev

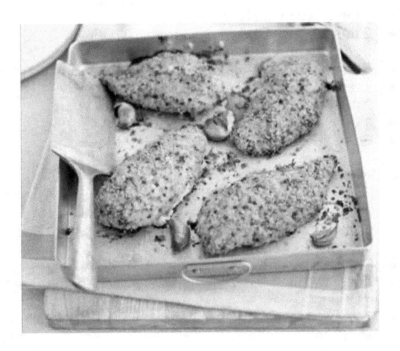

Prep Time: 25 minutes
Cook Time: 35
Servings: 4 people

Ingredients

- 6 minced garlic cloves
- ½ cup of the finely chopped parsley
- 1 cup of the breadcrumbs
- 4 skinless and boneless chicken breasts
- 2 tablespoons of the minced ginger
- 1 tablespoon of the mixed herbs to sprinkle
- 4 tablespoons of extra virgin olive oil

Directions

- Preheat an oven at 450 degrees
- Take a food processor, minced ginger, parsley, olive oil, some salt, black pepper and breadcrumbs. Pulse them until well combined and pulsed then put them in the plate
- Cut the slits in the chicken breast
- Then press the cheese into each hole and press the edges to seal
- Spread the olive oil on the chicken breasts and press the Herby crumbs onto them
- Then put the coated chicken in the baking pan. Sprinkle some minced garlic around the chicken then drizzle some olive oil
- Then let then bake for about 25 minutes until the chicken is cooked and the breadcrumbs is turned into golden brown
- Then squeeze the soft and roasted garlic
- The serve them and enjoy

Ultimate Chorizo Ciabatta

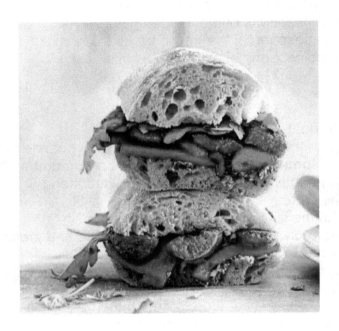

Prep Time: 5 minutes
Cook Time: 15 minutes
Servings: 2 people

Ingredients

- 2 cups of the ciabatta
- 2 cups of the packed and cooking chorizo cut into halves sized or lengthwise
- 1 cup of pesto
- 1 cup of the roasted red pepper
- Handful of the rockets
- Some salt to taste
- Some ground black pepper to taste

Directions

- Preheat an oven at 450 degrees F
- Take out the griddle pan on medium heat, then put the ciabatta to heat up
- Then put the chorizo for 5 minutes. Until they are cooked and charred
- Let them open the warm ciabatta, then spread them pesto, then make a layer of the red peppers. Then heat up chorizo. Then put the rocket, then put the ciabatta together. Then cut them in two halves
- Then serve them and enjoy

Baked Teriyaki Pork And Veggies

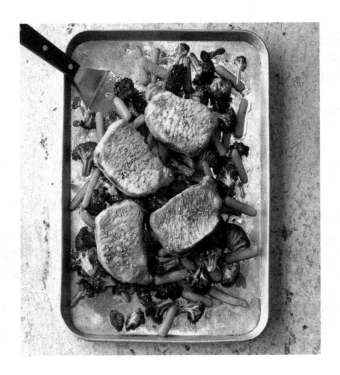

Prep Time: 15 minutes
Cook Time: 30 minutes
Servings: 4 people

Ingredients

- 2 cups of the hand torn broccoli florets
- 1 cup of the baby carrots halved or lengthwise
- 1 tablespoon of the extra virgin olive oil
- 1 tablespoons of the freshly minced ginger root
- Some salt to taste
- Some ground black pepper to taste
- 4 boneless and skinless pork loin chops
- 5 tablespoons of the sodium-reduced teriyaki sauce
- 1 teaspoon of the toasted sesame seeds

Directions

- Preheat an oven at 450 degrees F
- Take a baking tray lined with foil spread the broccoli florets and carrots then sprinkle the peppers, olive oil, ginger, some salt and black pepper to taste toss them and make a single layer
- Then put the pork chops on the veggies. Drizzle the teriyaki sauce and let them bake for about 30 minutes until they are tendered or turned into golden brown
- Then remove them and top them with sesame seeds

Shortcut Oven-baked Chicken Chimichangas

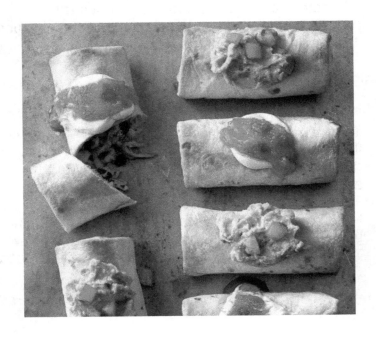

Prep Time: 15 minutes
Cook Time: 30 minutes
Servings: 6 people

Ingredients

- ¼ cup of the extra virgin olive oil
- 1 small sized onion finely chopped
- 3 cups of the rotisserie chicken cooked and shredded
- 1 package of the ready to serve rice
- 15 ounces of the black beans rinsed and drained
- 4 ounces of the chopped green chillies
- 3 tablespoons of the minced chipotle peppers dipped in adobo sauce
- ½ teaspoon of the cumin powder
- Some salt to taste
- Some ground black pepper to taste
- 2 cups of the shredded Mexican cheese blend
- ½ cup of the chopped fresh cilantro
- 10 inches of 6 corn tortillas (heat up)
- Some salsa to serve

Directions

- Preheating oven t 425 degrees F
- Place the baking tray in an oven
- Take a nonstick sauteing pan add some of the olive oil let it heat up then add the onions, let then sauté until they turned into golden brown and crispy
- Then add the chicken rice, beans, chipotle pepper, chiles, salt, ground black pepper, cumin powder
- Let them cook until they are cooked through
- Then remove them from the heat and stir in them some cheese and cilantro
- Now warm up the tortillas and spoon the mixture in each tortilla then let them fold. Repeat this process with the rest of the tortillas
- Then take a baking tray brush them with some olive oil then brush the olive oil on the tortillas
- Then transfer the pan to the oven and let them bake for about 15 minutes by flipping from both sides
- Then serve them with salsa and enjoy

Pizza Noodles Bake

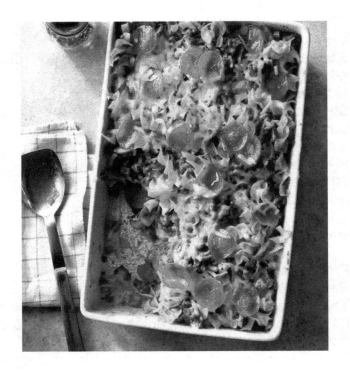

Prep Time: 25 minutes
Cook Time: 15 minutes
Servings: 6 people

Ingredients

- 10 ounces of the cooked egg noodles
- 2 pounds of the ground beef
- 1 small sized onion finely chopped
- ½ cup of the finely chopped green peppers
- 15 ounces of the pizza sauce
- 4 ounces of the mushrooms stems and pieces drained
- 1 cup of the shredded mozzarella cheese
- 1 cup of the cheddar cheese
- 4 ounces of the sliced pepperonis

Directions

- Preheat an oven at 425 degrees
- Then cook the noodles according to the package instructions.
- Meanwhile take a nonstick sauteing pan, add the olive oil, let the minced beef cook, then add the onion and green peppers on medium heat. Let them cook until it turns into golden brown and meat turns into crumbles then drain them and add pizza sauce and mushrooms
- Then let them heat through
- Now take a baking dish drainer half of the noodles and then make layers of minced beef, then cheese and pepperonis
- Then repeat these layers
- Let then cover and bake for about 20 minutes until they are heated through
- Then remove them from the oven and then serve them and enjoy

Cornbread Taco Bake

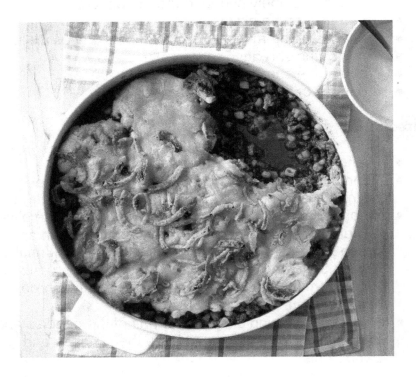

Prep Time: 20 minutes
Cook Time: 35 minutes
Servings: 8 people

Ingredients

- 2 pounds of the ground beef
- 14 ounces of the sweet corn kernels drained
- 1 can of tomato sauce
- ½ cup of the water
- ½ cup of the chopped green peppers
- ½ cup of the Taco seasoning
- 8 ounces of the cornbread mix
- 3 ounces of the french-fried onions divided
- ½ cup of the shredded mozzarella cheese

Directions

- Take a nonstick skillet add the extra virgin olive oil then add the minced beef let them cook on medium flame until no longer remains pink
- Then drain them and stir them in the water, corn kernels, and tomato sauce, taco seasoning and green peppers
- Then sprinkle some salt and black pepper to taste
- Then spoon them in the baking dish
- Now prepare the cornbread mixture according to the package directions and then stir in the french fried onions. Then spread them over the beef mixture
- Then transfer them to the baking oven at 425 degrees F and let them bake for about 20 minutes
- Then sprinkle on them cheese and remaining cheese and remaining onions. Let them bake for about 5 minutes until the cheese starts melting and bubbling
- Then serve them and enjoy

Tomato Basil Baked Fish

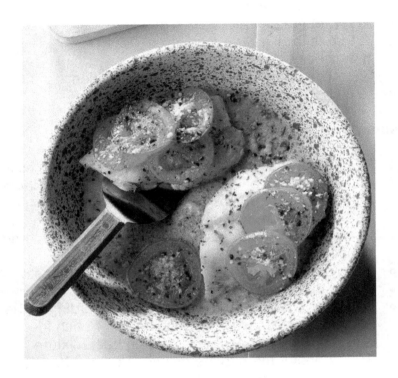

Prep Time: 10 minutes
Cook Time: 20 minutes
Servings: 4 people

Ingredients

- 1 tablespoon of the lemon juice
- 1 tablespoon of the extra virgin olive oil
- 8 ounces of red snapper cod, and haddock fillets
- ½ teaspoon of the dried basil leaves
- Some salt to taste
- Some ground black pepper to taste
- 2 plum tomatoes thinly sliced
- ⅛ cup of the grated Parmesan cheese

Directions

- Take a shallow bowl, add the lemon juice, oil, then add the fish fillets, then coat. Place them in the oil greased pie plate
- Then sprinkle with basil leaves, some salt and black pepper to taste
- Scatter the sliced tomatoes on the top. Then sprinkle with the cheese and the rest of the seasonings
- Then let them bake for about 450 degrees F for about 20 minutes until the fish become tendered and softened
- Then serve them and enjoy

Turkey Biscuit Skillet

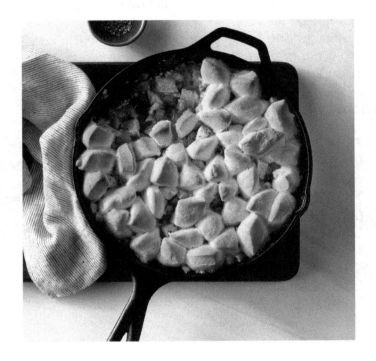

Prep Time: 10 minutes
Cook Time: 20 minutes
Servings: 6 people

Ingredients

- 1 tablespoon of the unsalted melted butter
- 1 small sized chopped onions
- ¼ cup of the all purpose flour
- 2 cups of the chicken broth (undiluted)
- ¼ cup of milk
- ½ teaspoon of red pepper
- 3 cups of the cube sized turkey breasts
- 2 cups of the frozen peas and carrots, thawed
- 12 ounces of the buttermilk biscuits

Directions

- Preheat an oven at 450 degrees F
- Take an ovenproof skillet and add some melted butter. Then add the onions let them sauté for about 4 minutes until they are softened and golden brown
- Take a bowl add flour, broth, milk, and pepper stir them to combine until they are well combined
- Then stir them in the pan, let them boil while stirring occasionally. Let them cook for about 2 minutes. Then add the turkey and frozen vegetables. Let them heat through
- Then arrange the biscuits on the top. Transfer them to the oven and let them bake for about 20 minutes until they are turned into golden brown
- Then serve them and enjoy

Potato And Pepper Sausage Bake

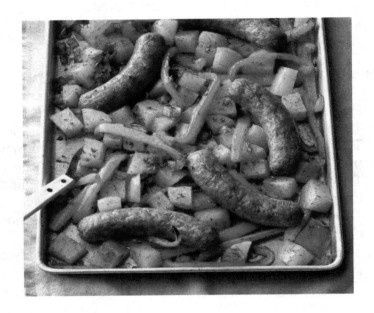

Prep Time: 25 minutes
Cook Time: 30 minutes
Servings: 5 people

Ingredients

- 5 large sized Yukon potatoes peeled and cut them in cube shaped
- 1 large sweet orange pepper thinly sliced
- 1 large sweet red pepper thinly sliced
- 1 shallot finely chopped
- 4 minced garlic cloves
- 1 tablespoon of extra virgin olive oil
- 2 tablespoons of the smoked paprika
- Some salt to taste
- 1 teaspoon of the dried thyme
- 1 teaspoon of the red pepper
- 19 ounces of the sausage links
- Some finely minced thyme leaves to garnish

Directions

- Preheat an oven at 450 degrees F
- Take a baking pan, put the potatoes, sweet peppers oil, salt, pepper, shallots and garlic. Toss them to coat well
- Spread them evenly on the pan. Then put the sausages
- Transfer them to the baking oven and let them bake for about 35 minutes until they sausages are softened and tendered
- Sprinkle some chopped thyme leaves then serve them and enjoy

Basil Butter Steaks With Roasted Potatoes

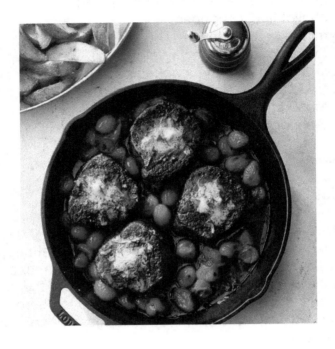

Prep Time: 10 minutes
Cook Time: 20 minutes
Servings: 4 people

Ingredients

- 16 ounces of the frozen Parmesan and roasted garlic red potatoes wedges
- 4 beef tenderloin steaks
- Some salt to taste
- Some ground black pepper to taste
- 5 tablespoons of the unsalted melted butter
- 2 cups of the grape tomatoes
- 1 tablespoon of the freshly minced basil leaves

Directions

- Preheat an oven at 450 degrees F
- Bake the potatoes wedges according to the package directions
- Take a bowl add the streaks sprinkle some salt and black pepper, let them coat and then put them in an ovenproof skillet
- Drizzle some butter and let them bake for about 20 minutes
- Then a bowl add the add the basil leaves and butter, then spoon them over the steaks and then serve with potatoes
- Then serve them and enjoy

Sliced Ham With Roasted Vegetables

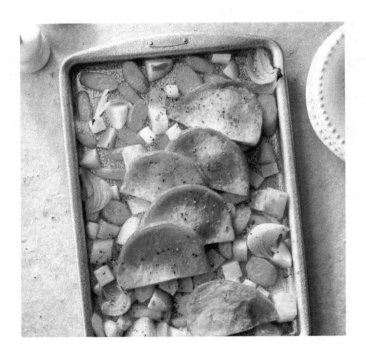

Prep Time: 10 minutes
Cook Time: 35 minutes
Servings: 6 people

Ingredients

- 1 teaspoon of the extra virgin olive oil
- 7 potatoes peeled and cut them in diced form
- 5 medium-sized carrots thinly sliced
- 1 medium-sized turnip peeled and cut into cube sized
- 1 large sized onions, cut then into wedges
- 6 ounces of the cooked ham cut them in thin slices
- 5 tablespoons of the thawed orange juice
- 3 teaspoons of the brown sugar
- 1 tablespoon of the prepared horseradish
- 1 tablespoon of the grated orange zest
- 1 teaspoon of the coarsely ground black pepper

Directions

- Preheat an oven at 450 degrees F
- Grease the baking pan, with some olive oil
- Then add the potatoes, turnip, carrots, and onion
- Drizzle some olive oil
- Transfer the baking pan to the oven and let them bake for about 30 minutes
- Then remove them and put the sliced of the ham over the vegetables
- Now take a bowl add the horseradish, brown sugar, and orange zest. Pour this over the ham and veggies and then let them bake for about 10 minutes. Then sprinkle with the pepper

Nutty Barley Bake

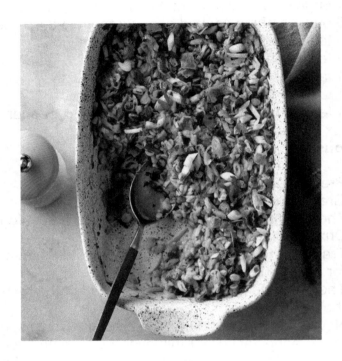

Prep Time: 15 minutes
Cook Time: 1 hour minutes
Servings: 5 people

Ingredients

- 1 medium sized chopped onions
- 1 medium-sized cup of pearl barley
- ½ cup of the slivered almonds
- ¼ cup of the butter cut them in cube sized
- ¼ cup of the chopped parsley
- ¼ cup of the thinly sliced green onions
- Some salt and black pepper to taste
- 2 cans of the beef broth
- Some chopped parsley and green onions to garnish

Directions

- Preheat an oven at 459 degrees F
- Take a nonstick sauteing pan add the butter and then put the onions and let them sauté for about 3 minutes until they are tendered or turned into golden
- Then add the barley and nuts in them. Then stir in them greens onions, parsley, some salt and black pepper
- Let them stir and then put them in the oil greased pan. Then stir in the beef broth. Let them bake for about 1 hour until the liquid is absorbed
- Then sprinkle some finely chopped parsley and green onions

Baking Appetizers

Bacon Wrapped Jalapenos

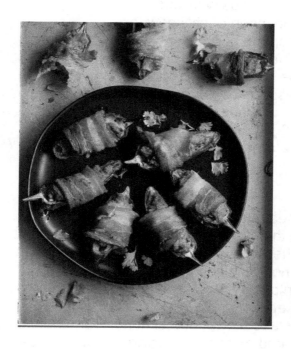

Prep Time: 5 minutes
Cook Time: 15 minutes
Servings: 2 people

Ingredients

- 3 cups of almond flour
- ½ cup of chopped cilantro
- 1 large onion chopped
- 2 golden eggs whisked
- 2 tablespoon of chili powder
- 1 teaspoon of paprika
- ½ tablespoon of cumin powder
- Some kosher salt to taste
- 1 teaspoon of chipotle powder
- 1 lbs. of ground turkey
- 10-12 jalapenos pepper
- 10-12 slices of bacon

Directions

- Preheat the oven at 400 degrees F
- Line the air fryer basket with the parchment paper
- Preheat the jalapenos peppers cut them in lengthwise (Remove the seeds from the peppers)
- Then place the jalapenos peppers on the air fryer basket
- Now take a bowl add almond flour, chopped cilantro, chopped onions, chili powder, paprika powder, cumin powder, salt and chipotle powder
- Stir them together and then add the minced turkey in it
- Take one tablespoon of turkey mixture in the jalapenos pepper. Wrap the bacon slices in each pepper.
- Place the toothpick to secure. Now place the jalapenos peppers to their fryer basket. Cook them in the air fryer basket for 15 minutes
- Serve them with ranch dip

Rivoli

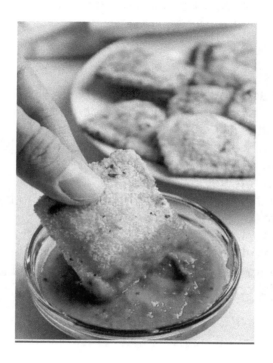

Prep Time: 15 minutes
Cook Time: 15 minutes
Servings: 2 people

Ingredients

- 15 frozen rivoli
- 1 cup of buttermilk
- 1 cup of breadcrumbs
- Marina sauce for dipping or any of your favorite sauce
- Olive oil for spraying

Directions

- Preheat an oven at 370 degrees F
- Take 2 bowls one for the breadcrumbs and second for the buttermilk
- Dip each piece of rivoli in the buttermilk mixture and then in the breadcrumb's mixture.
- Coat them well
- Place this rivoli in the air fryer basket and bake it for 7 minutes
- After 4 minutes spray some olive oil on the top of the rivoli an then place it in the air fryer basket and bake it for 3 minutes more than remove them and serve with your favorite sauce or Marina sauce
- Enjoy

Crab Cakes

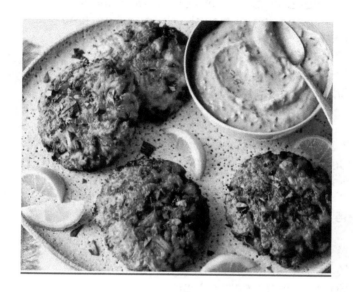

Prep Time: 10 minutes
Cook Time: 25 minutes
Servings: 4 people

Ingredients

- 2 golden eggs
- ¼ cup of mayonnaise
- ½ cell peppers finely chopped
- 3 tablespoons of fresh chopped chives
- 3 tablespoons of freshly chopped parsley
- 1 tablespoons of lemon juice
- 3 tablespoons of Dijon mustard
- 2 tablespoons of fish seasoning
- Some kosher salt to taste
- Some ground black pepper to taste
- 1 pound of crab meat
- 3 cups of panko breadcrumbs
- Cooking oil for spraying
- Some lemon wedges for serving

Chipotle Sauce

- ½ cup of mayonnaise
- ½ cup of sour cream
- Some kosher salt to taste
- Some ground black pepper to taste
- Some chopped fresh parsley
- Some chopped chives
- 2 tablespoons of adobo sauce

Directions

- Take a bowl, crack the eggs, whisk them together until well combined, add mayonnaise, bell peppers, chives, parsley, lemon juice, mustard sauce, seafood seasonings, some kosher salt, some ground black pepper. Mix all the ingredients together by using your hands
- Then cover the bowl with a plastic cover and set it aside for 1 hours
- For the chipotle sauce.

(Whisk together the mayonnaise mixture, sour cream, adobe sauce, chipotle, chives, parsley and lemon juice, whisk them together until well combined. Season them with salt and black pepper

- Now make crab patties by using your hands and give them round shape
- Preheat an oven at 370 degrees F and then spray the air fryer basket. Place the patties inside the air fryer basket and top with some cooking oil
- Cook them for 16 minutes and then serve them with the chipotle sauce and lemon wedges
- Enjoy

Lemon Pepper Wings

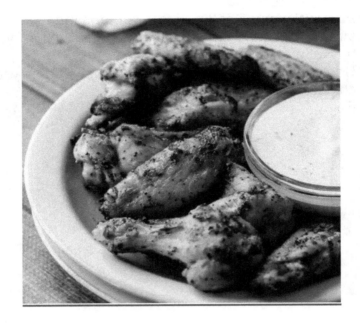

Prep Time: 10 minutes
Cook Time: 35 minutes
Servings: 8 people

Ingredients

- 1 lbs. of chicken wings (Tips Discarded)
- 3 tablespoons of lemon pepper seasonings
- Some kosher salt to taste

Directions

- Preheat an oven at 400 degrees F before 5 minutes
- Take a large bowl add chicken wings
- Then add lemon pepper seasonings
- Sprinkle some salt
- Toss the ingredients together until well combined for 4 minutes and let it marinate for 1 hour
- Then place these chicken wings in the air fryer basket and cook them for 10 minutes
- Then serve with favorite dipping sauce
- Enjoy

Zucchini Chips

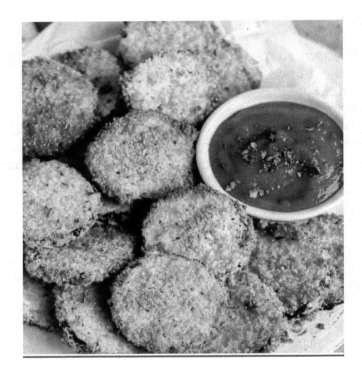

Prep Time: 10 minutes
Cook Time: 15 minutes
Servings: 8 people

Ingredients

- 2 cups of panko breadcrumbs
- 3 tablespoons of cornmeal
- ⅓ cup of grated Parmesan cheese
- ½ tablespoon of dried basil
- ½ tablespoon of dried oregano
- ⅛ teaspoon of cayenne pepper
- 1 cup of zucchini cut into slices
- 1 golden egg beaten

Directions

- Preheat an oven at 350 degrees F
- Take a bowl crack golden egg beaten them
- Now take another bowl add breadcrumbs, cornmeal, dried basil, dried oregano, cayenne pepper and Parmesan cheese mix all the ingredients together until well combined
- Dip each slice of zucchini in the egg mixture and then in the breadcrumbs mixture
- Repeat this process with the rest of the slices then place this in the air fryer basket and cook it for about 5 minutes
- Then serve with your favorite sauce and enjoy

Air Fryer Loaded Tater Tots

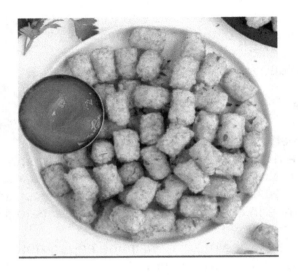

Prep Time: 10 minutes
Cook Time: 20 minutes
Servings: 9 people

Ingredients

- 17 ounces of frozen tater tots
- Cooking oil for spraying
- Marina sauce for dipping

Directions

- Preheat an oven at 370 degrees F
- Spray with some cooking oil
- Place the tater tots in the basket and cook it for about 7 minutes until it turns golden brown and crispy
- After that remove from the basket and serve it with your favorite sauce or Marina sauce and enjoy

Air Fryer Cinnamon Sugar Dessert Fries

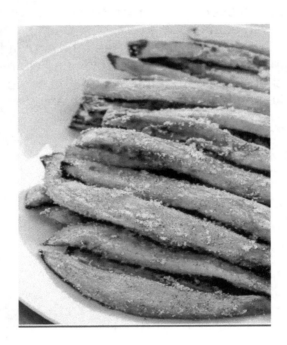

Prep Time: 10 minutes
Cook Time: 15 minutes
Servings: 6 people

Ingredients

- 2 sweet potatoes thinly sliced
- 2 tablespoons of melted butter
- 1 tablespoon of melted butter (Keep it separated from the above)
- 2 tablespoons of sugar
- ⅓ tablespoon of cinnamon
- Some kosher salt to taste
- Some ground black pepper to taste

Directions

- Preheat an oven at 370 degrees F
- Take a bowl add peeled and thinly sliced sweet potatoes
- Pour 1 tablespoon of melted butter coat them
- Cook the fries in the air fryer basket for about 15 minutes
- Remove the fries from the air fryer basket and place them in the bowl
- Coat them with the remaining butter and pour the sugar and cinnamon
- Toss them to coat the fries
- Serve them with your favorite sauce and enjoy

Air Fryer Frozen Onion Rings

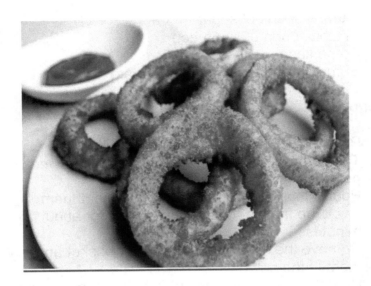

Prep Time: 10 minutes
Cook Time: 15 minutes
Servings: 2 people

Ingredients

- 7 ounces of frozen onion rings
- Some marina sauce for dipping
- Extra virgin olive oil for spraying

Directions

- Preheat an oven at 370 degrees F
- Spray with some extra virgin olive oil
- Place the onion rings in the air fryer basket and cook it for about 7 minutes
- Remove from the basket and serve with your favorite sauce or Marina sauce
- Enjoy

Air Fryer Hamburgers

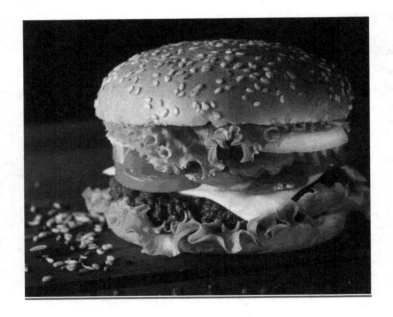

Prep Time: 10 minutes
Cook Time: 25 minutes
Servings: 1 people

Ingredients

- 1 pack of frozen hamburger patties
- 2 cabbage leaves
- Sliced tomatoes as desired
- 2 cheese slices
- Chilli sauce as desired
- 2 buns for burger

Directions

- Preheat an oven at 370 degrees F
- Spray the basket with non stick cooking spray
- Place the hamburger patties in the air fryer basket and let them cook for about 10 minutes by flipping them halfway through
- Now take buns place the cabbage leaves on the bun
- Then put the cooked patties then cheese slice, and sliced tomatoes spread some chili sauce again place the cheese slices and cabbage leave put the bun on them and serve it with ketchup and enjoy

Frozen Mozzarella Sticks

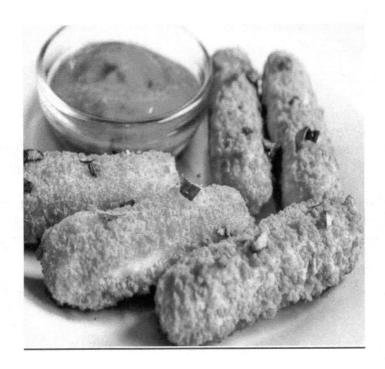

Prep Time: 10 minutes
Cook Time: 25 minutes
Servings: 5 people

Ingredients

- 12 frozen mozzarella sticks
- Any of your favorite sauce for dipping
- Finely chopped fresh parsley
- Olive oil for spraying

Directions

- Preheat an oven at 370 degrees F
- Spray with some extra virgin olive oil
- Then place the mozzarella cheese sticks in the basket. Cook it for 10 minutes
- You can check after 10 minutes if the cheese inside the sticks are softened
- After that remove from the air fryer basket and serve with Marina sauce and enjoy

Conclusion

Thank you, my readers, for making it to the end! Following the recipe instructions from this cookbook to maintain your results and live a healthy and happy life.